LIZ EARLE'S
QUICK GUIDES
Antioxidants

B⬛XTREE

Advice to the Reader

*Before following any advice contained in this book, it is
recommended that you consult your doctor if you suffer from any health
problems or special condition or are in any doubt.*

First published in Great Britain in 1995 by Boxtree Limited,
Broadwall House, 21 Broadwall, London SE1 9PL

10 9 8 7 6 5 4 3 2 1

ISBN: 0 7522 1663 5

Text design by Blackjacks
Cover design by Hammond Hammond

Printed and bound in Great Britain by
BPC Paperbacks Ltd

A CIP catalogue entry for this book is available from
the British Library

Contents

ACKNOWLEDGEMENTS

I am grateful to Sarah Hamilton Fleming for helping to produce this book. Also to Professor Anthony Diplock and Dr Michael Hertog for supplying valuable research material. I am also indebted to the talented team at Boxtree, Rosemary Sandberg and Claire Bowles Publicity for their unfailing enthusiasm and support.

Introduction

The last few years have witnessed a revolution in nutritional thinking. We now know that there is a link between diet and many kinds of serious disease. The antioxidant nutrients have emerged as some of the most powerful weapons we have in the fight against heart disease, cancer and even the ageing process. Young or old, it is never too late to benefit from the many benefits these special nutrients can bring. This *Quick Guide* gives you all the scientific and medical evidence, together with an update on the latest research from around the world.

Liz Earle

1

Antioxidants in Action

In recent years a few molecules – beta-carotene, vitamin C and vitamin E – have been causing quite a stir in the world of science and medicine. These, and other nutrients, act as antioxidants, which means that they have the potential to keep us healthier and younger for longer. Scientists made these exciting new discoveries when they began to investigate more closely the link between diet and the likelihood of developing certain diseases. One of the major results of these studies is in showing that people in countries where the diet is rich in fruit and vegetables are less likely to develop heart disease and many forms of cancer. Further investigation has suggested that this is due to the high level of antioxidant vitamins and minerals in fruit and vegetables.

Today, the majority of health problems are caused by degenerative diseases. It has been discovered that the antioxidants found in fruit and vegetables and certain herbs can help prevent many of these illnesses. Beta-carotene (the vegetable form of vitamin A), vitamins C and E, selenium, copper, zinc, manganese and other nutrients are all antioxidant, which means that they not only improve our well-being, but they also protect every cell in our body. Each year more antioxidants are discovered and top-level research around the world shows that these vital nutrients are so powerful that they provide us with the potential to boost our immunity against life-threatening illnesses, prevent serious disorders, such as cataracts, and even reduce the signs of ageing.

Antioxidants are present in many types of food and occur naturally. They are safe substances to take in normal amounts, to maintain and encourage better health. Unfortunately, the same cannot be said of many prescription drugs, and there is increasing concern over the use and efficacy of many of our common modern-day drugs. All drugs have side-effects but, more importantly, research is revealing that many of the so-called 'wonder drugs' simply do not live up to their original promise.

Studies show that the use of supplements is 1,000 times safer than drugs. In a five-year period the only report of a fatality due to taking vitamin supplements reported by American poison control centres was later found to be incorrect. By contrast, during the same period, drugs of all kinds caused over 1,000 deaths (excluding the figure for suicide by overdose). The toxicity of the key antioxidant vitamins (A in the form of beta-carotene, C and E) is particularly low.

The Free Radicals

Human beings need oxygen to survive – the body uses oxygen to derive energy from food in order to fuel bodily processes. Oxygen is moved around the body by haemoglobin, which contains iron (this is why our blood is dark red). Thanks to haemoglobin, our blood can absorb fifty times more oxygen than water. Oxygen is carried in the bloodstream throughout the body to feed all our living cells. The process of converting oxygen into energy is called oxidation and is essential for life.

There is, however, a serious side-effect: the process of oxidation creates *free radicals* which can harm us by damaging our cells. Free radicals are constantly being created within the body; while you are reading these words they are being mass-produced inside you. Although a certain amount of free-radical activity is needed by our bodies to kill bacteria, an excess quickly causes problems.

Free radicals are largely a by-product of oxidation. When the body burns food to make energy, it also burns germs and toxic substances such as ozone and carbon monoxide. These small fires give off 'sparks', or highly active free radicals. These damage the delicate membrane that surrounds our cells, disturb chromosomes and genetic material and destroy valuable enzymes, causing a chain-reaction of damage throughout the body. Research suggests that free radicals are a major contributory factor in at least fifty of our most prevalent diseases, including coronary heart disease, lung disease, certain cancers, cataracts, rheumatoid arthritis, Parkinson's disease and even the ageing process itself.

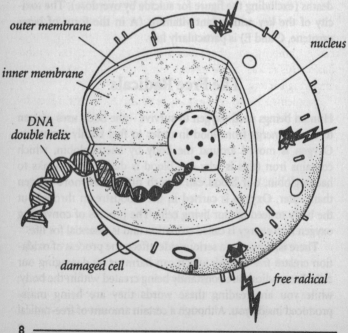

outer membrane

nucleus

inner membrane

DNA
double helix

damaged cell

free radical

To appreciate fully the damage free radicals cause it is worth taking a quick chemistry lesson. Free radicals are molecular fragments with an unpaired electron. Unfortunately, electrons are friendly creatures and prefer to go around in pairs. So the free radicals try to 'grab' another electron from a passing molecule. A free radical is, therefore, a loose-living electron playing the field for a mate to settle down with. It will break up other pairs to find a partner, and create many more unstable molecules in the process. In short, a chain reaction occurs within the body which damages our cells.

Not all free radicals are damaging and a few are useful in boosting our immune system. Some enzymes need free radicals in order to function properly, and they are also needed to expand our blood vessels and keep blood flowing freely around the body. Free radicals are required to kill germs and help the white blood cells in our immune system fight bacteria. This can be seen when we cut or graze our skin and a certain amount of inflammation appears before the wound heals. This reddish swelling is due to the action of free radicals attacking bacteria.

Problems arise when the body produces too many free radicals and the process gets out of control. It is the *balance* of free radicals, rather than the particles themselves, that is important.

The Danger from Increased Exposure

As we have seen, free radicals are produced by oxidation: the same process that causes butter to go rancid when it is left out of the fridge or cars to go rusty when exposed to the air. Although the body doesn't go rancid or rusty, its cells are affected in a similar way, which is why free radicals are so damaging. They are continually being produced within the body as an important component of our normal metabolism. In an ideal world, free radicals would be dealt with by our in-built safety mechanisms.

They are also created by a number of external agents, such as pollution, which is rapidly spreading in our environment. Increasing exposure to factors such as pesticides, tobacco smoke, car exhaust fumes and ultra-violet radiation (from ozone depletion) adds up to more free radicals being created than the body can cope with. The world we live in has changed dramatically over time, and this change has brought with it exposure to many more free radicals in the form of pollution and a highly processed diet.

DNA and Free-Radical Damage

All life on earth, from grass to gorillas, is built around the genetic information carried within DNA, which are quite simply the most important (and the most complex) molecules in the world. The scientifically minded will know that the acronym stands for deoxyribonucleic acid. All the messages of heredity are carried within DNA, which ensures that generations of living things continue to grow as they always have done. One human DNA molecule contains enough information to fill over 3,000 books the size of this title, and DNA molecules are present in every cell in our bodies.

DNA resembles two chains twisted together to form a spiral or double helix. Genetic messages are written along these spirals in the form of chemicals known as 'base pairs' which join the double helix together like the steps of a spiral staircase. When cells divide and multiply, the double helix splits and each chain carries an identical set of genetic material to two new cells.

Free radicals damage DNA by attacking the sugars and phosphates that form the backbone of the double helix. Once these are damaged, DNA cannot give the correct instructions to make protein. This leads to mutations and the creation of substances within the body which shouldn't be there.

Excess free radicals affect the body at its most basic level. They can attack and infiltrate every living cell. The prime targets of free radicals are the fats, or lipids, that make up our cell walls. This type of attack is referred to as lipid peroxidation, meaning that the fats have been altered by oxidation. One of the leading experts on free radicals, Dr Catherine Rice-Evans, Director of the Free Radical Research Group based at Guy's Medical School in London, explains:

Inside the cell walls are various components that are doing different set tasks within the body. Free radicals attack the lipids and damage the cell membrane, causing these components to leak out. You can compare this to an egg with a damaged or broken shell – its contents leak out and make a mess. These components of the cell usually behave very well when they are inside their membrane, but when they escape and get to be somewhere they shouldn't, they become damaging. The important point about free radicals is the chain reaction of damage that they cause, which is responsible for the premature death of a cell or the alteration of its response to hormones and neurotransmitters. Free-radical damage also prevents enzymes from regulating all bodily reactions and can even cause the mutations of our cells that lead to cancer.

The Antioxidant Answer

Antioxidants can be used to fight against excess free radicals, neutralising and preventing them from causing more damage within the body. Antioxidants have the ability to transform free radicals into less dangerous substances. Studies based on large groups have shown beyond doubt that low levels of beta-carotene and vitamins C and E lead to high levels of disease.

2

How to Avoid
Free Radicals

High levels of free radicals in our bodies are predominantly caused by pollutants in the atmosphere. Many health organisations have expressed concern over the rising levels of free radicals. The UK Ministry of Agriculture, Fisheries and Food is certainly taking the issue very seriously and is funding extensive projects at the Free Radical Research Unit.

Poisoned by Pollutants

When we breathe in polluted air or tobacco smoke we are inhaling one of the most potent sources of free radicals. Although we cannot always see or smell them, many noxious substances, including carbon monoxide, nitrogen dioxide and lead from car exhausts, pollute the air we breathe. This remains an ongoing problem in the industrialised world. Over half the population of America and a large proportion of people in Europe are currently breathing in toxins at levels that far exceed US Environmental Protection Agency 'ambient air quality' standards.

In addition to car fumes, we are surrounded by many other invisible poisons. These include industrial pollutants such as cadmium, mercury and lead, which escape into the atmosphere as by-products of industries such as battery manufacturing, mining, smelting and metal working. Toxic hydrocarbons are also released by processes like paint spraying, dry cleaning, printing, oil refining, and plastics and chemical manufacturing.

Ground-level ozone is now a serious problem for many smog-filled cities. Although ozone protects the earth when it is high in the sky, ground-level ozone is poisonous if directly inhaled, causing eye, nose and throat irritation and damaging the lungs. High levels of ozone also trigger asthma attacks.

Our lungs are the first major body tissues that these airborne toxins encounter. Inhaled toxins are also especially damaging because they proceed straight from the lungs to the rest of the body without passing through any detoxification process. Lung tissue is particularly vulnerable because it comes into direct contact with these noxious substances as they are breathed in, and the cell walls in our lungs are extremely thin and delicate.

Once inside the lungs, the free radicals thus produced assault the enzymes that enable our lungs to expand and contract. Without this elasticity, we find it hard to breathe and are unable to take in all the oxygen we need. In smokers, this can be seen in the disease called emphysema. These inhaled pollutants also destroy red blood cells and damage our immune system.

Airborne pollution is extremely hard to avoid and it is impractical to suggest that we leave our homes and jobs in the cities or the suburbs and move to a cleaner environment in, say, the Outer Hebrides. Fortunately the antioxidant vitamins and minerals offer us some useful protection from the effects of pollution. This is particularly important for children, who have been shown to be especially at risk from long-term exposure to pollutants because they have a higher metabolic rate and breathe in more air than adults. It is, therefore, essential to make sure that children receive adequate supplies of antioxidants in their diet.

A study reported in the *American Journal of Clinical Nutrition* in 1991 showed that vitamin E is helpful in protecting us against the effects of ozone in smog. But studies have also shown that city dwellers have lower levels of antioxidant vitamins in their blood. Beta-carotene, vitamin C and vitamin E are needed throughout the body for many functions, but when we breathe in polluted air these are used up in the battle to fight free radicals. This leaves the rest of the body dangerously low in supplies. If we run out of antioxidant nutrients, free radicals take over and a state known as 'oxidative stress' occurs, leaving free radicals 'free' to cause damage throughout the body.

Stub it Out!

It has been estimated that, in industrialised countries, tobacco is now causing about 2 million deaths a year, killing at least a third of those who regularly smoke cigarettes. Smoking a cigarette is equivalent to force-feeding the body with free radicals. Cigarette, cigar and pipe smoke contain over forty known cancer-causing compounds, including carbon monoxide, hydrogen cyanide, nitrogen dioxide and cadmium. Smoking tobacco also causes an increase in our own inflammatory cells, which are themselves potent producers of free radicals.

Smoking damages passive smokers as well. The burning end of a cigarette produces nitrogen dioxide, a powerful free radical, which can be inhaled by the non-smoker. Studies have shown that the spouse of a heavy smoker is more than three times as likely to develop lung cancer than the spouse of a non-smoker. Children are particularly at risk, as the free radicals they inhale damage their developing tissues. Dr William Cahan, a specialist in lung cancer at the Memorial Sloan–Kettering Cancer Centre in the US, bluntly states that 'Parents who smoke in the presence of their children are committing child abuse.'

It seems there is no end to the long list of damage caused by smoking. There is increasing evidence that smokers and passive smokers alike need higher levels of beta-carotene, vitamin C and vitamin E in their diet to combat the damage being done.

Cigarette smokers have lower levels of vitamin C in their bloodstream than non-smokers: in a recent American study, it was found that smokers needed to consume at least 150mg of vitamin C a day (the amount found in four fresh oranges) in order to achieve blood levels of the vitamin comparable to those found in non-smokers. Other more conservative figures estimate that smokers need 70–80mg a day more vitamin C than non-smokers.

Vitamin C is an important component in collagen, which keeps our complexion supple, which may be one reason why studies at the Wilson Dermatology Clinic in North Carolina have found that smokers have many more facial lines and wrinkles than non-smokers. Other studies show that levels of beta-carotene are also low in smokers. One survey revealed that those who smoked a packet of cigarettes a day had 25 percent less beta-carotene in their blood than non-smokers, despite consuming the same amount in their food.

Radiation Risks

Radiation is a general term which refers to energy waves, or electro-magnetic radiation (EMR). The wavelength determines the type of radiation, eg light waves, radio waves, or microwaves. In terms of free-radical production, the most potent forms of radiation are nuclear energy, X-ray and ultra-violet (UV). Normally, one doesn't encounter the first two in a large degree, but UV radiation is all around us.

Television screens, VDUs, computers and other electrical installations all produce EMR at fairly low levels. They also emit a magnetic field, which creates static but has a less certain link with free radicals. However, there is some evidence to suggest that electro-magnetic fields do 'encourage' free radicals, even though the subject of electro-magnetism and free radicals is very much a speculative area of research.

Dr Keith McLauchlan, a leading researcher in the field of physical chemistry at Hertford College, Oxford, suggests that there is a possible link between electricity and free radicals. His research has shown that free radicals respond to electro-magnetic fields such as those emanating from power lines. Thus, more free radicals may be produced, increasing the probability of damage.

DYING FOR A TAN?

The sun's rays give us light and warmth. The sun also emits UV radiation: the two main wavebands are called UVA and UVB. Even on a cloudy day we receive doses of both UVA and UVB radiation through our skin. In moderation, this radiation is essential to life. In excess, whether in one dose or by continued exposure, it is extremely harmful.

UVA constitutes about 80 percent of all the UV radiation we are exposed to. UVA rays not only hit the surface of the skin – they pass straight through the upper layers and reach the dermis below. Down in the dermis the UVA rays destroy the supporting collagen and elastin fibres of the skin as well as generating free radicals. UVA radiation is the main cause of premature skin ageing. Although UVA sunbeds probably won't give you skin cancer, they might make your skin sag!

UVB rays account for about 20 percent of the radiation we are exposed to. This waveband is mainly absorbed in the upper layer of the skin where it stimulates the production of the brown pigment called melanin, which gives us our sun tan. Too much UVB radiation causes the skin to redden and burn. UVB rays also damage the DNA in cells and are the main cause of skin cancer, as large numbers of free radicals are generated.

Malignant melanoma is the most serious form of skin cancer and it is increasingly common. Dr Rice-Evans confirms that 'melanoma is a direct result of free-radical action on the skin from a radiation source. Those most at risk have naturally pale skins, ie the north European races.' Some types of skin cancer can be fatal. In fact, deaths due to skin cancer have been doubling every decade.

SKIN CANCER RISKS

The rate of skin cancer is rising rapidly, partly because we tend to spend more time in the sun and partly because of the diminishing of the ozone layer that shields us from the worst of the sun's rays. There is now such a large hole in the ozone layer above Australia that two out of three Australians will have suffered some form of skin cancer by the age of seventy-five. Unfortunately, skin scientists are predicting similar problems for Britain. The ozone layer has reduced by at least 8 percent over Europe and it is estimated that, by the year 2000, the ozone layer will have reduced by 30 percent. Any reduction in the ozone layer inevitably means more radiation on the ground below. In turn, this results in more free radicals being formed inside the body.

A simple way to remember the effects of UV radiation on the skin is that UVA rays mainly cause **Ageing** and UVB rays mainly cause **Burning**.

Alcohol

We all know that excessive drinking of alcohol is bad for us. Alcohol is not only a powerfully addictive drug, but too much also leads to large numbers of free radicals being produced in the liver.

In the midst of all this bad news, however, it is cheering to learn that moderate amounts of alcohol may actually be good for us! Red wine, in particular, has been found to contain powerful antioxidant substances that can neutralise free radicals. These antioxidants come from substances called procyanadins, found in grape skins. Procyanadins are found only in red wine because the vinification process involves the grape skins being left in contact with the wine to give it colour. The red wine grape also contains the beneficial antioxidant compounds known as flavonoids (see Chapter 5).

However, as almost all grapes are heavily sprayed with fungicides which are themselves free-radical producing, one should choose organic varieties of red wine. As with all things, though, moderation is the key.

In heavy drinkers, alcohol, as well as drugs such as paracetamol, can interact with normal liver biochemistry to produce free radicals which damage the liver tissues. This is believed to be the cause of cirrhosis of the liver and liver failure. All dietary studies involving heavy drinkers have also found disturbingly low levels of vitamin C, thought to be caused by bad eating habits and the fact that alcohol prevents the metabolism of vitamin C.

Free Radicals in Food

We are increasingly at risk from free radicals in our food. Fats, such as cooking oils, are the main source of these deadly molecular monsters. As fats are heated, their chemical structure starts to break down, forming peroxides. These, in turn, break down to form the hydroxyl radical. This type of free radical is highly reactive and causes a great deal of damage to our cells and DNA. Professor Diplock, who is at the forefront of antioxidant research in the UK, explains that: 'when our DNA is attacked in this way it causes mutagenesis which may then go on to cause cancer'. The occasional fry-up won't kill us, but eating fried foods regularly over twenty or thirty years may well build up enough altered, toxic products within the body to affect our basic biochemistry and lead to disease.

Polyunsaturated fats such as sunflower and safflower oil are the least stable at high temperatures. These become 'oxidised' more quickly than monounsaturated fats, such as olive oil. The best option when frying foods, therefore, is to use olive oil. Dr Rice-Evans explains that: 'an oil will oxidise if it has two or more double bonds in its chemical structure (such as polyunsaturated oils). As olive oil only has one double bond it is much more stable when cooking. It is the only vegetable oil I use in my kitchen.'

The lipid peroxidation that occurs when heating a cooking oil can be prevented by vitamin E, in which vegetable oils are naturally rich. The exact vitamin E content depends on how much the oil has been tampered with. Unrefined corn oil, for example, has plenty of vitamin E to prevent peroxidation, but when it is refined and stripped of its natural constituents to produce a light, clear oil it loses at least a third of its natural vitamin E. In general, pale, clear, cooking oils have the least vitamin E and are the most susceptible to peroxidation. The same is also true of low-fat spreads and margarines made from highly refined oils. Some manufacturers recognise this problem and are starting to put vitamin E back into their products, although unfortunately they often add synthetic vitamin E which is not as potent as the natural variety. The answer is to buy unrefined and cold-pressed oils.

All oils need careful storage. Polyunsaturated oils such as sunflower and safflower are broken down by heat and light, so they are best kept in a cool cupboard. Olive oil is more robust and may be kept at room temperature. It is important that all oils are stored in a dark place, as light will spoil oil extremely quickly – a good example of EMR (electromagnetic radiation) at work.

Because oils oxidise when exposed to air, they should also be kept tightly sealed. It is better to buy cooking oils in small quantities and replace them frequently to prevent this happening.

ALTERED FOOD STATES

Although monounsaturated vegetable oils are believed to be healthy, some oils can become damaging when they are processed. Trans-fatty acids are artificially created in food processing when natural fats are chemically altered. Trans-fatty acids are principally produced during the process of hydrogenation, whereby a liquid vegetable oil is hardened through the use of hydrogen gas to make a solid fat. Hydrogenation allows cheap cooking oil to be turned into a semi-solid or hard fat with a long shelf life. These fats are a primary constituent of margarines and low-fat spreads, and are very widely used, eg in making cakes, biscuits, crackers, sweets and other processed foods. You may even find hydrogenated vegetable oil in vitamin pills!

This process of hydrogenation and the creation of trans-fats is a special cause for concern as it may be linked to heart disease. A recent study carried out by researchers at the Harvard Medical School, and published in *The Lancet*, connects trans-fatty acids to an increase in coronary heart disease. The study involved 85,000 women over a five-year period; when their intake of trans-fatty acids was analysed, there emerged a clear relationship between high levels of these fats and high rates of heart disease.

Some foods, such as toast, or barbecued meats, are burned in the cooking process. This burning produces large numbers of free radicals. The long-term implications of this are unknown, and the odd piece of burnt toast is unlikely to do much harm, but charred foods should not be eaten too often.

Salt-cured and salt-pickled (brine) foods have been linked to cancer as they contain nitrates. These are acted on by free radicals to create nitrosamines, which are among the most carcinogenic substances known. Fortunately, the formation of nitrosamines is prevented by antioxidants.

High levels of other nitrates in our drinking water cause a problem. Nitrates can be turned into nitrites by certain bacteria and fungi and have been shown to be strongly linked to cancer. In recent years the levels of nitrates in our drinking water have greatly increased because they are used as agricultural fertilisers. They then leach out into rivers and streams and end up in our tap water. The EU limit for nitrates in drinking water is fifty parts-per-million (ppm) although, for many years, several water authorities have exceeded this. Some types of water filter will reduce the levels of nitrates in tap water, or you can buy bottled water that specifies a low nitrate level. This precaution also reduces other sources of free-radical activity in our water supply, such as chlorine and pesticides.

Genetics

Heredity plays an important part in many diseases and it has been said that we should choose our parents carefully! The genetic material that we inherit from our parents is an integral part of all our cells and plays an important part in our pattern of health. Obviously, we cannot alter our genetic make-up, but once we know where our genetic weakness lies, we can protect ourselves from diseases to which we may be susceptible. For example, if there is a history of heart disease in your family it is prudent to avoid smoking, cut down on the amount of saturated fat you eat and increase your intake of vitamin E. Likewise, if there have been cases of certain cancers in your family, eating plenty of foods rich in beta-carotene should help to boost your protection.

The Causes of Free Radicals

The list below shows how exposed to free radicals you can be in your daily life.

* Living in or close to a city.

* Living near industrial sites such as chemical factories or power stations.
* Living near a main road or motorway.
* Driving in traffic.
* Working with toxic chemicals, eg dry-cleaning chemicals, photographic chemicals, etc.
* Smoking.
* Spending long hours in front of the television or a computer screen.
* Using a microwave oven.
* Spending long hours exposed to the sun.
* Not wearing sunscreens.
* Eating too many fried foods.
* Eating too many processed foods.
* Eating too much barbecued food.
* Drinking more than three units of alcohol a day if you are a man or more than two units a day if you are a woman.
* Not eating enough fruit and vegetables (five servings a day, ideally).

If you find that many of the above are true for you then beware! You need to watch what you eat and increase your consumption of fresh fruit and vegetables – aim for at least five portions of fruit or vegetables every day. It may be worth considering taking supplements of the antioxidant nutrients if you find it difficult to achieve this. There are many combinations of these nutrients available in tablets or capsules from chemists and health food shops.

Antioxidants are also added to many foods as natural preservatives. For example, vitamin E is added to some fats and oils to delay rancidity and vitamin C is used as an 'improver' to make the gluten in white bread more elastic, producing a softer loaf. Antioxidants can be identified on food labels as follows:

* Vitamin E is listed as E306–E309. Natural vitamin E is E306; E307, E308 and E309 are all synthetic forms of vitamin E
* Vitamin C is listed as E300–E304. It may also be called ascorbic acid.

We all have different levels of excess free radicals within us, depending on stress, diet and lifestyle. For this reason, we do not all need the same amount of antioxidants in our diet. The Free Radical Research Group is now looking into the benefits of personalised levels of antioxidants to fit individual needs. This has been promoted by the work of Dr Bruce Ames, a molecular biologist at the University of California. He believes that the idea of a 'recommended daily allowance' for antioxidant vitamins is outdated. Dr Ames has developed a test to measure antioxidant levels in the blood so that, if someone's levels are low, or their oxidised fats are high, they can be put on a stronger antioxidant diet than a person whose antioxidant levels are in balance. Catherine Rice-Evans says: 'No two people absorb or deplete nutrients at the same rate. If individuals could be prescribed personal antioxidants, this would be much more effective in promoting longevity.' Perhaps in years to come antioxidant tests may be as easily available as blood tests.

3

The Antioxidant Vitamins

Vitamins are involved in many body processes; if we don't get enough of them, we can become ill and even die of vitamin deficiency. The antioxidant vitamins also have extra powers: beta-carotene (precursor to vitamin A), vitamin C and vitamin E can effectively combat free radicals. These vital vitamins fight against the effects of oxidation, and scientists are now recognising the importance of this when it comes to preventing degenerative diseases.

We can see the results of oxidation all around us in everyday life. For example, if you slice up an apple and leave it for half an hour, the flesh quickly turns brown because the apple is reacting with oxygen in the air. An identical process is taking place within our own bodies every second of our lives. Although we can't see what's going on, our body is literally 'rusting' from within, due to this continual process of oxidation and the action of free radicals. You can't stop oxidation, because it is a part of the life process, but you *can* deal with the side-effects.

The antioxidant nutrients that help to keep us youthful, fit and healthy are nature's answer to the damage caused by oxidation. Each of these nutrients works in a slightly different way, but the overall effect is to mop up the free radicals as they form and prevent them from doing serious damage within the body. As free radicals are continually created, it is well worth maintaining high levels of each of these vital vitamins.

Beta-carotene

It is important not to confuse beta-carotene with vitamin A as the two are separate substances. One source of vitamin A is foods that derive from animals, such as meat and milk, and this is called *retinol*. The other source of vitamin A is the *carotenoids* – found in fruit and vegetables. There are more than 600 varieties of carotenoids, although the only one of these of which we have a great deal of knowledge is beta-carotene. The body is able to convert beta-carotene into vitamin A as it needs it, so it is a very safe version of this nutrient. Large amounts of vitamin A are toxic, whereas the same amount of beta-carotene is totally safe.

Beta-carotene is a natural plant dye and was first discovered in carrots, hence the name given to the entire family. The carotenoids are a colourful range of pigments that provide the huge variety of colours that we see in nature. Scientists first became interested in them over 150 years ago when, in the 1830s, researchers looking into the biology of plants pin-pointed the yellow pigment, that gives autumn leaves their colour, as being the carotenoid called lutein. Around fifty of the 600 carotenoids which have been identified since then can be converted by the body into vitamin A, but beta-carotene is by far the most effective. It is stored in the body in fatty tissues and the liver, and a small amount also circulates in the bloodstream.

Beta-carotene itself is a deep shade of reddish-orange and is the main pigment in yellow and orange fruit and vegetables. Foods rich in beta-carotene, such as carrots, stand out on the supermarket shelves because of their bright colours. The riper the produce, the more beta-carotene it will contain. Dark green leafy vegetables such as spinach and broccoli also contain high levels of beta-carotene, although they are a different colour because the green chlorophyll pigment is more dominant. As a general rule, the darker or more vivid the colour of the fruit or vegetable, the more beta-carotene it will contain. For example, lollo rosso lettuce leaves contain more beta-carotene than the pale iceberg variety.

The role of beta-carotene in plants is to help prevent fruits and vegetables from burning in the sun, in the same way that we release melanin which turns the skin brown and protects our skin against sun damage. Free radicals are formed in plants, just as in humans, by UV radiation; nature provides the antidote in the form of beta-carotene, which shields the plant from radiation. Human beings also gain some sun protection from eating up their greens on a regular basis. Studies by Professor Micheline Matthews-Roth of the Harvard Medical School show that beta-carotene helps humans whose skin is overly sensitive to sunlight. Professor Matthews-Roth has spent over twenty years studying the effects of beta-carotene on the skin and, as a result, the powerful US Food and Drug Administration (FDA) has approved it for the specific treatment of light-sensitive disorders. Beta-carotene has also been tried out on other types of sun-sensitivity, such as prickly heat, and supplements for these disorders are now available on prescription in America.

Although beta-carotene is non-toxic and safe to take in large quantities, it can have the peculiar side-effect of turning the skin orange! This is caused by the pigment temporarily staining the skin from within. Taking mega-doses of beta-carotene, say 300mg daily, is a cheap way of obtaining a fake suntan.

There are two kinds of beta-carotene supplements: natural and synthetic. The natural beta-carotene pills are more expensive, and are pretty similar to the beta-carotene found in food. Man-made beta-carotene supplements are derived from petro-chemicals and contain higher levels of trans-fats (see Chapter 2).

Natural beta-carotene has lower levels of these unwanted trans-fats and is boosted by other members of the carotenoid family, such as lutein and alpha-carotene, which are also antioxidants. The natural beta-carotene found in supplements does not come from an obvious source, such as carrots, but from an unusual type of marine algae, *Dunaliella salina*. Algae are extremely efficient at manufacturing beta-carotene to protect themselves from the sun's rays. When choosing a natural beta-carotene supplement, look for the words 'natural source' or 'natural *D. salina* beta-carotene' on the label.

THE ANTI-CANCER PILL?

Apart from the welcome benefits of protecting the skin and discouraging wrinkles, the most important discovery concerning beta-carotene has been in the field of cancer. This devastating disease currently kills more than 160,000 UK citizens every year and touches every family in the land, as one in three of us are affected by cancer at some point in our lives and one in five people in the UK will die from it. While the medical profession continues its search for a cure, recent research suggests that preventing the disease in the first place may be a far easier option. Although no one knows exactly how or why cancer strikes, it is evident that those who eat the most beta-carotene also have the lowest rates of certain cancers. Numerous nutrition studies conducted on large populations have found that the risk of lung cancer and cancers of the stomach, oesophagus and cervix are all lower in those who eat plenty of beta-carotene. The same cannot be said of vitamin A, which suggests that it is the unusually powerful antioxidant quality of beta-carotene that has an anti-cancer effect.

Scientists now believe that eating an abundance of fresh fruit and vegetables will provide sufficient beta-carotene to give significant protection against cancer. Although the existing evidence is limited, it has sparked major trials involving beta-carotene. The evidence for a protective effect is particularly strong in the case of lung cancer. Thirty out of thirty-two epidemiological studies included in a recent review showed that a reduced risk of developing lung cancer is linked to high intakes of fresh fruit and vegetables. There have been more than forty studies into the beneficial effects of beta-carotene on cancer, involving tens of thousands of people world-wide.

DAILY ALLOWANCE

Beta-carotene is measured in micrograms (mcg or µg) and milligrams (mg). There are 1,000mcg to 1mg. Some studies suggest that we should be aiming for a minimum of 15,000mcg (15mg) a day. This level can only be achieved in our diet by eating *at least* five generous portions of fruit and vegetables a day.

THE OTHER CAROTENOIDS

In contrast to beta-carotene, very little is yet known about the effects of most of the other carotenoids. Scientists have known about carotenoids for the last fifty years, but they were only interested initially in their role as precursors to vitamin A. It is only very recently that scientists have discovered their antioxidant properties.

Researchers at the University of Hawaii have recently re-analysed a study of the relationship between diet and lung cancer using new information on the composition of five carotenoids. The carotenoids they looked at were alpha-carotene, beta-carotene, lutein, lycopene and beta-cryptoxanthin. These carotenoids, along with zeaxanthin, can be found in at least 120 different fruits and vegetables. The study involved 230 men and 102 women with lung cancer and 597 men and 268 women from the general population, who were matched for age and sex. The researchers discovered that beta-carotene, alpha-carotene and lutein each demonstrated protective effects against lung cancer depending on dosage. The effects of all three carotenoids were of similar magnitude. It is interesting to note, however, that the protective effect of eating vegetables was stronger than the effects of the three carotenoids alone, which suggests that other components of vegetables also contribute to cancer prevention. This is one reason why it is best to get the antioxidants we need from their natural source, ie fruit and vegetables, as these contain a unique blend of nutrients which is impossible to imitate synthetically.

Professor Thurnham of the Human Nutrition Research Group at the University of Ulster is another expert on carotenoids and is particularly interested in the antioxidant activity of lutein. His studies appear to show that lutein and some of the other xanthophyll carotenoids are more successful than beta-carotene in reducing free radicals. Some studies even suggest that these carotenoids are more efficient than vitamin E.

Lycopene is another rising star in carotenoid research. Lycopene is the red pigment in tomatoes, red peppers and watermelon. Researchers at the University of Illinois measured the blood-carotenoid levels of 102 women with a pre-cancerous inflammation of the cervix known as CIN (cervical intraepithelial neoplasia) and questioned them about their dietary habits. The testing was repeated for 102 similar, disease-free, women. The analyses showed that the women with the highest blood levels of lycopene had five times less risk of developing CIN than those with the lowest levels of the carotenoid. A simple answer for better health may be to eat more tomatoes!

THE CAROTENOID COMPOSITION OF FOODS

The Institute of Food Research, in Britain, has recently developed and evaluated a method for the analysis of carotenoids in fruit and vegetables. The levels of carotenoids in the different parts of the fruits and vegetables tested varied considerably, and the nation's intake of carotenoids depends upon the individual's preference for certain items, seasonal availability and the amount of fruit or vegetables that are eaten. For example, the carotenoid analysis of selected commonly consumed items indicates that watercress, spinach, broccoli, peas, green peppers, beans, lettuce and Brussels sprouts are potentially good sources of lutein. However, spinach and watercress are eaten by relatively small numbers in the population. Peas are the main source of lutein for most people while tomatoes are the main source of lycopene. Carrots provide over 70 percent of beta-carotene intake, although the vegetables which are a good source of lutein are also good sources of beta-carotene. Fruits do not account for much of the intake of lutein, lycopene or beta-carotene, although they are the main source of beta-cryptoxanthin.

Unlike the other antioxidant vitamins, the carotenoid content of foods is little affected by cooking methods and there is even some evidence to suggest that cooking increases the 'bioavailability' of carotenoids to humans. Bioavailability is a term used to describe how easy it is for our bodies to make use of the nutrients we get through our diet.

Vitamin C

Vitamin C is probably the best-known of all vitamins and it is the one many of us turn to when attempting to ward off the common cold. This amazing vitamin possesses many extraordinary properties, but the bottom line is that it is absolutely essential for keeping us alive. If we are not getting enough vitamin C in the diet then we are at risk from infections and can even die from scurvy. Unlike other nutrients, vitamin C has a strong social history as the result of this disease. In the seventeenth and eighteenth centuries scurvy was a common cause of death among sailors at sea for months on end, living on a somewhat unbalanced diet of salted meat, ship's biscuit and rum. It was not uncommon for a ship to lose more than half its crew to scurvy, just because of a lack of vitamin C. Scurvy was not confined to the navy and has appeared throughout history at times of food shortages, such as during

siege warfare. It affected rich and poor alike, and some histori-
ans believe it killed Henry VIII, who was notorious for his
dislike of fruit and vegetables. Records show he lived almost
entirely on meat and sugary puddings, and this lack of vitamin
C could have been the cause of his swollen limbs, leg ulcers,
blotchy skin and extreme irritability.

Chemically speaking, vitamin C is one of the simplest vitamins, which is why it was among the first to be studied. Yet,
although it was officially identified over seventy years ago,
scientists are still discovering fascinating new ways in which it
works. Its basic function is to help with the growth and repair of
body tissues and to help maintain healthy gums, blood vessels,
bones and teeth. It also boosts the immune system and may
help the body fight off bacterial and viral infections.

The body also needs vitamin C to make collagen, the
biological glue that sticks our cells together. Low levels of
vitamin C in the body can lead to low levels of collagen and
this reduces the elasticity of our lung tissue, so that the lungs
are not able to function properly. This is one plausible reason
why elderly people with insufficient vitamin C intake are more
likely to suffer from respiratory ailments such as bronchitis
and pneumonia.

Vitamin C is also one of the antioxidant nutrients and so
fights the formation of free radicals. Unlike beta-carotene,
vitamin C is water-soluble, and is therefore found in the fluids
between our cells. Vitamin C acts as a roaming agent, fighting
the free radicals that cross its path as it travels throughout the
body. It is not stored in the system, so we need to eat foods that
are rich in vitamin C every day to maintain a constant supply. It
is impossible to take too much vitamin C as any excess simply
passes through the body and is excreted in urine. The only side-
effect of taking large quantities of vitamin C (upwards of
2,000mg, or 2g, daily) might be mild diarrhoea. Indeed, high
doses of vitamin C have been used as a natural laxative!

It has been rumoured that vitamin C contributes to kidney stones because it is metabolised using oxalic acid, a substance implicated in the formation of kidney stones. However, there is no clear evidence of such a link, even with mega-doses of the vitamin. Nevertheless, commonsense advice for anyone suffering from kidney problems is to avoid high doses of vitamin C.

THE BIOFLAVONOIDS

In vitamin supplements, the natural form of vitamin C comes from either acerola cherries or corn and is most effective when combined with bioflavonoids – a group of colouring pigments that top up a plant's antioxidant protection against environmental stresses. Supplements that combine vitamin C with bioflavonoids are known as vitamin C complex. Bioflavonoids are needed to strengthen the network of the capillary blood vessels that run throughout the body; they are especially important for the appearance of our skin and work in tandem with vitamin C to strengthen capillary walls and prevent bruising. If you are prone to developing broken blood vessels near the surface of your skin, then a diet rich in bioflavonoids will help to strengthen your skin and prevent this occurring. All the fruits and vegetables that contain vitamin C are also a good source of bioflavonoids.

These water-soluble nutrients occur in tiny quantities and cannot be stored in the body, which is why eating a regular supply of fresh foods is so important in order to maintain correct levels of vitamin C and bioflavonoids. A diet that is high in fresh fruit and vegetables typically provides a total of 1,000–2,000mg (1–2g) per day of the whole range of bioflavonoids. The best sources are apricots, blackcurrants, broccoli, Brussels sprouts, cherries, citrus fruits, grapes, green peppers, guavas, kale, parsley, strawberries, tomatoes and watercress.

Research into the bioflavonoids is in its infancy but is already turning up some interesting findings. For example, it is believed that, by reinforcing cell membranes, bioflavonoids may help prevent the leakage of excess antibodies in the bloodstream of allergy sufferers. Certain bioflavonoids have also been found to block the production of inflammatory agents called leukotrienes in the body. As these are the foremost biochemical cause of asthmatic symptoms, the potential for using bioflavonoids to treat fever, asthma and other allergies is exciting. Some bioflavonoids are also highly antioxidant (see Chapter 5).

VITAMIN C AND CANCER

Studies have shown that people who eat more vitamin C have a reduced risk of cancer. More than forty studies have been conducted on the relationship between vitamin C and cancer. According to Professor Gladys Block, nutrition specialist at the National Cancer Institute in the US, the evidence for the protective effect of vitamin C against cancers of the oesophagus, larynx and oral cavity is 'strong and consistent'. There is also less consistent evidence that vitamin C protects against cancers of the cervix, colon, stomach and pancreas. In addition, a study by researchers at the University of California has found that those who consume high levels of vitamin C live longer generally and are particularly protected from heart disease. This is possibly because vitamin C works in unison with vitamin E, which has also been shown to help reduce the risk of heart disease.

DAILY ALLOWANCE

Vitamin C is usually measured in milligrams (mg) or grams (g). 1,000mg is equal to 1g. The recommended daily allowance (RDA) for adults in Britain is currently 40mg, although the new European recommendation is 60mg and many experts suggest this should be raised to at least 100mg.

COOKING TIPS

As vitamin C is destroyed by heat, fruit and vegetables are best eaten either raw or very lightly cooked. Of all the vitamins, it is vitamin C that disappears most quickly during cooking. This is because it is water-soluble and dissolves into the cooking water. It is, therefore, better to steam vegetables or cook them in the microwave in order to preserve their content of vitamin C. As much as 75 percent of the vitamins in green vegetables can be lost by simmering. Vegetables such as broccoli and cauliflower are best placed directly into boiling water. This is because the oxidising enzymes that destroy vitamin C do not work at high temperatures – they are most effective at around 60–85°C and so, by putting vegetables in cold water and bringing them to the boil, we destroy most of the vitamin. Use a minimum of water, as vegetables that are completely immersed lose up to 80 percent of their vitamin C. If they are just one-quarter covered they lose half as much of this essential vitamin.

When cooking vegetables in water don't throw the vitamin C down the sink after draining; use it as a nutritious base for soups, sauces, stock or gravy. Cooking vegetables in a copper or iron pan should also be avoided as these metals react with vitamin C and destroy it.

Over-cooking is another major cause of vitamin loss: approximately 25 percent of vitamin C is lost after fifteen minutes of cooking, compared to 75 percent after 90 minutes of cooking. Vitamin C escapes from food when it is exposed to the air, eg after it has been cut, chopped or crushed. Food processing such as canning and bottling also reduces the vitamin C content of foods, particularly in fruits that contain dark red pigments.

In addition, storage time affects vitamin content. While freshly dug raw potatoes have around 30mg of vitamin C per 100g in October, this will have dropped to 8mg by the following March. The key is to buy fresh fruit and vegetables when they are in season so that they will not have been sitting in storage for months on end. This will add a bit of variety to meals, as with each season you will be eating a completely new range of fruit and vegetables. However, this is not as easy as it sounds; modern food retailing usually involves the supply of 'fresh' fruit and vegetables all year round. Try consulting a kitchen-gardening book to brush-up on natural seasonal availability.

This loss also applies to fruit juices: apple juice loses half its vitamin C after four to eight days in the fridge; orange squash loses up to half its vitamin C content within a week of opening the bottle, and after three months it may have lost it all. Shaking the bottle or carton of juice mixes in more oxygen and so destroys the vitamin C even faster.

Vitamin E

Vitamin E is possibly the most important free radical fighter because it protects every cell in the body. The term vitamin E was first used in 1922 to describe a substance discovered in vegetable oils that was essential to maintaining fertility in rats. In 1936, an American research scientist, Dr Evans, isolated the most potent form of natural vitamin E from wheatgerm oil and analysed its chemical structure. The term vitamin E actually applies to a whole family of chemical compounds called tocopherols, of which d-alpha tocopherol is the most effective.

Since its discovery, vitamin E has been nicknamed the 'virility vitamin' because it plays such an important part in human fertility. However, this is the least of its powers: it is also essential for maintaining a healthy immune system as it strengthens white blood cells against infection and has particularly strong links with preventing heart disease. A study by the World Health Organisation identified low levels of vitamin E as being the single most important risk factor in death from heart disease

– more important even than high cholesterol, raised blood pressure or smoking. The other remarkable attributes of vitamin E include the ability to dissolve blood clots, strengthen blood capillary walls, improve the action of insulin in diabetics, increase muscle power and clean up pollution in our internal system. Vitamin E also influences hormonal processes, reduces the severity of inflammations and plays an important part in anti-ageing skincare products.

If you are not getting enough vitamin E in your diet, your health can be seriously impaired. Loss of vitamin E can lead to the loss of red blood cells, muscle wastage and sterility. The signs of deficiency are not obvious as there is no specific disease caused by insufficient amounts of the nutrient. The effects of too little vitamin E in our daily diet usually develop over long periods of time, and are linked with many degenerative disorders including premature ageing and arthritis.

Vitamin E is fat-soluble and is, therefore, found in fatty tissues of the body including the protective membrane of our cells. In humans, vitamin E is stored in the areas of the body that need it most, including the heart, muscles, testes, uterus, blood, and the adrenal and pituitary glands. Extra supplies are also tucked away in the liver for future use. Vitamin E is an extremely safe nutrient and it is virtually impossible to store too much of it.

The most exciting aspect of this powerful vitamin is that it is considered to be the single most important antioxidant nutrient. It works by preventing the oxidation of fats, hence its vitally important function in safeguarding the layer of protective fatty tissue which surrounds all our internal cells and major organs. The more polyunsaturates we eat, such as those in sunflower oil spreads, the more vitamin E we need to consume. Some brands of margarine add vitamin E to their products so look out for this on the labels. Vitamin E works in partnership with vitamin C to neutralise free radicals as they are formed.

NATURAL VITAMIN E IS BEST

Vitamin E is found in the oils of vegetables, pulses and seeds such as wheatgerm, sunflower, corn, peanut and rapeseed. These all contain d-alpha tocopherol which is the 'single' form of vitamin E. Synthetic vitamin E is made from eight different substances, only one of which has the same molecular make-up as natural vitamin E. The synthetic variety is produced from petrochemicals and is officially recognised as being 36 percent less effective than natural vitamin E. Recent trials suggest that natural vitamin E is more likely to be **twice** as effective as its synthetic counterpart. If you decide to take a supplement of vitamin E, do make sure that it is the natural variety. Many brands now state that they contain natural source vitamin E. Alternatively, you can recognise the type of vitamin E by the letter 'd', as in d-alpha tocopherol. Synthetic vitamin E begins with a 'dl', as in dl-alpha tocopherol.

Natural foods rich in vitamin E comprise vegetable oils (particularly wheatgerm oil), seeds, nuts and wholegrains. Fish oil is also high in the vitamin.

VITAMIN E FOR A HEALTHY HEART

Vitamin E has hit the headlines as a result of exciting research that shows we can reduce our risk of heart disease with natural vitamin E supplements. Data published in the *New England Journal of Medicine* in June 1993, involved over 87,000 nurses. Harvard University researchers observed a protective effect in those taking a daily supplement of more than 100iu (international units) of vitamin E a day. No such results were observed in those who adjusted their diet to include more vitamin E-rich foods. Those who had taken vitamin E supplements for two or more years had half the risk of heart disease of those who had not taken the supplement.

This finding is extremely significant, and has resulted in greater studies being carried out to determine if we all should be taking a daily dose of vitamin E to maintain a healthy heart. Another study of almost 40,000 American male health professionals also supports a strong association between a high intake of vitamin E and a low risk of coronary heart disease. Interestingly, this time the researchers could not find such a link with vitamin C and a lower risk of heart disease, and beta-carotene was only found to be beneficial with smokers and former smokers. It may be that vitamin E is our most powerful antioxidant ally in the fight against heart disease.

DAILY ALLOWANCE

Vitamin E should be measured in milligrams (mg), but international units (iu) may also be given. 1mg of natural vitamin E (d-alpha tocopherol) is equivalent to 1.49iu. At present, there is no RDA for vitamin E in Britain, although the European guidelines recommend 10mg daily. However, much of the recent research into vitamin E and disease prevention has involved considerably larger doses.

COOKING TIPS

Vitamin E is found mainly in vegetable oils, nuts and wholegrains such as wheat. Unfortunately, any type of processing of wholegrains reduces their vitamin E content. Oatmeal loses only a little as just the hull is removed from the grain, but the refining of white flour leads to 92 percent of the original vitamin E being lost from the wheat. This is why white bread has so little vitamin E in comparison to brown wholemeal.

Valuable vitamin E supplies are also broken down by oxygen. A bottle of safflower oil stored at room temperature for three months will lose more than half its vitamin E content. This loss increases if the oil is stored in a warm, light place such as a sunny shelf or window-sill. The best way to preserve the vitamin E content of all foods, including cooking oils, is to store them in a cool, dark larder.

Cooking also significantly reduces the amount of vitamin E in food. Deep fat frying and deep freezing are the main culprits. Frying food can destroy up to 90 percent of the vitamin E content.

This vital vitamin has also been shown to block the formation of cancer-causing nitrosamines which are created by a reaction between free radicals and nitrites present in smoked, pickled or cured foods. So if you insist on eating smoked bacon make sure you fry the rashers in a vegetable oil that is rich in vitamin E. Better still, marinate the bacon beforehand in such an oil and then grill it.

4

The Antioxidant Minerals

Vitamins are not the only 'good guys' in the battle against free radicals: there is a whole group of antioxidant minerals. In fact, the body's first line of defence in fighting the damage caused by free radicals comes from a group of enzymes that contain the minerals manganese, copper, zinc and selenium. Enzymes control all the chemical changes which take place in our cells, including the creation and release of the energy that is life itself. Enzymes are catalysts: they assist chemical processes, but they must be triggered into action by certain minerals before they can work.

Manganese

This element is found in tiny quantities in water, plants, animals and humans. The human body contains around 12–20mg of manganese in total, most of this being deposited in the bones, pancreas and liver. However, we lose some of our manganese supply every day through the process of excretion, so we need to acquire regular amounts from our diet. Manganese has many functions within the body and helps to regulate our growth and maintain a healthy nervous system, bone development and brain functioning. It is also an essential part of the genetic code contained within all our cells. Manganese is a component of the enzyme superoxide dismatase (SOD for short!). This enzyme has the power to react with free radicals and deactivate them, rendering them harmless.

Manganese is principally found in wheatgerm. The husk is removed from wheat during refining, which is why white bread contains only one-sixth of the manganese found in wholemeal bread. Manganese is also present in tea, so if you are unable to go through the day without having at least five cups of tea, you will be getting useful amounts of manganese. Hazelnuts are another major source. Those eating a diet that is rich in wholegrains, nuts and seeds are unlikely to run short of manganese. Manganese is one of the safest minerals to add to the diet as any excess is simply excreted.

DAILY ALLOWANCE

Manganese is measured in milligrams (mg) and no RDA has yet been established in Britain. In America, the RDA for adults is between 2 and 5mg.

Copper

Copper is an essential element of life for humans, animals and most plants. Copper is all around us, in both the Earth's crust and the seas. Although it is vitally important, only tiny traces are needed in the body. For this reason it is known as a trace element. Copper is stored in our blood, bones and liver as well as being an important component of many enzymes, including SOD.

In addition to its antioxidant properties, copper also protects us from respiratory problems and infections, and is needed for the production of haemoglobin in our blood. Copper is a part of the skin proteins collagen and elastin and it is important for maintaining a clear, smooth complexion. It is also needed to make the pigment that colours our skin and hair. Copper is plentiful in many fresh foods, including wholegrains, beans, peas and green leafy vegetables and it is rare to suffer from copper deficiency, although this can be a cause of anaemia.

Many people who suffer from arthritis maintain that wearing a copper bracelet on their wrist reduces pain and inflammation of the joints. There is some medical evidence to support this, as traces of copper do dissolve in the skin's acid secretions and become absorbed into the bloodstream. Such additional copper supplies may help prevent arthritis from taking a hold and, in some cases, reduce the severity of the symptoms.

Copper deficiency, although rare, has been seen to occur in those who do not eat enough copper-rich foods such as nuts, wholegrain cereals, wholemeal bread and vegetables such as carrots. Vitamin C is known to interfere with the absorption of copper, so anyone taking high doses of vitamin C would be wise to balance this with a multi-mineral supplement that contains copper. Copper-rich foods include liver, crab, hazelnuts, lentils and olives.

DAILY ALLOWANCE

Copper is measured in milligrams (mg) and the RDA for the intake of copper in adults is 1.2mg. The National Research Council for Food and Nutrition in America recommend a daily intake of 1.5–3mg.

Zinc

Although we need only tiny amounts of zinc it is an essential mineral for maintaining good health. Zinc acts as a 'traffic controller' in the body, directing and overseeing the flow of body processes and the maintenance of our cells. It is found in tissues throughout the body and is an integral part of DNA. Zinc is needed to make both the male sperm and the female ovum. The developing foetus also requires zinc to ensure healthy bones, brain and nervous system. Zinc is important, too, for converting food into energy and it helps in the formation of insulin. It teams up with calcium to strengthen our bones and helps to prevent osteoporosis, or softening of the skeleton.

Zinc plays a part in the production of over eighty enzymes and hormones in the body, so it is not surprising that a lack of this mineral should have widespread effects. The body can store reasonable amounts of zinc, but it relies mainly on a regular intake in food. Too much zinc can cause nausea and fever, but too little will stunt growth and harm the immune system. The small number of cases of zinc poisoning are generally caused by industrial pollution.

As well as protecting us from within, zinc also makes an important contribution to keeping our skin smooth, supple and blemish-free. Studies by Dr Michaelson, of Uppsala University in Sweden, into the relationship between zinc and the skin have revealed that, in the treatment of a number of skin conditions, notably acne, prescribing zinc supplements can be as beneficial as some antibiotic treatments.

Low levels of zinc have been noted in disorders as diverse as acne, psoriasis, hyperactivity and schizophrenia. Many factors deplete the levels of zinc in the body, such as the contraceptive pill, steroid drugs, cigarettes and alcohol. Heavy smokers or drinkers, women taking the contraceptive pill, diabetics, pregnant and breastfeeding women should all consider taking a daily zinc supplement. It is also an important nutrient for teenagers as it promotes growth processes.

Zinc can be found in bread and other foods made from wheat such as pasta, but these also contain phytates which bind with minerals such as zinc making it difficult for the body to make use of it. For this reason other sources such as meat and vegetables are better foods for keeping our zinc levels high.

Liver, beef, pork, chicken, low-fat cheese, oily fish, shellfish and wholegrains are particularly high in zinc.

Vegans may be at risk of zinc deficiency as they do not eat meat, fish or dairy products and tend to have a greater intake of foods such as bread, pasta and textured vegetable protein (TVP), all of which contain high levels of phytates. Food refining strips zinc from our foods; brown rice contains six times as much zinc as the polished, white varieties. The level of zinc in the soil has also been systematically reduced over the years by intensive farming techniques, which has led to lower levels in crops, including wheat and root vegetables.

DAILY ALLOWANCE

Zinc is measured in milligrams (mg) and, as yet, there is no RDA in Britain. However, the European recommendation for zinc in adults is 15mg and studies in Britain show that our average daily intake is only around 10.5mg a day.

Selenium

Selenium is a silver-grey metal which was first identified in 1817 by two Swedish chemists. It is a giant in nutritional terms and has many functions within the body, including a role in protecting us from heart disease and cancer. Large doses of selenium are poisonous and it was only in 1957 that researchers at the University of California discovered the mineral's usefulness in preventing liver damage. Now selenium is recognised by scientists and nutritionists alike as being an essential part of our diet.

We need only tiny quantities of selenium, but it has many uses in the body. It keeps the liver functioning healthily, boosts the immune system by protecting our white blood cells, and maintains healthy eyes, skin, hair and heart performance. Selenium is a component of semen and plays an essential role in fertility. It also acts as one of the body's waste disposers, removing toxic cadmium and mercury from the body (essential if you are a smoker or breathe in other forms of polluted air). Perhaps most important of all, selenium is a vital component of the enzyme glutathione peroxidase, which helps to prevent damage from free radicals.

Selenium is an unusual mineral in that it boosts the powers of other vitamins within the system. When selenium is linked with vitamin E in the body, the vitamin lasts longer and is able to work harder. Selenium and vitamin E work synergistically, that is to say, they have a greater effect working together than they do separately. Protective enzymes produced in the body need both selenium and vitamin E to function effectively. In addition, studies on cancer in animals show that selenium increases the potency of vitamins C and E, and that this combination may give better relief from angina (chest pains) than using vitamin E on its own.

Vitamin E has an important role in protecting essential nutrients such as vitamin A, vitamin C, essential fatty acids and amino acids. It acts as an antioxidant in preventing these substances from breaking down and losing their strength, both in the food we eat and in the body. It is considered to be the most powerful antioxidant. Most good antioxidant supplements contain selenium as well as boost the protective effect of vitamin E.

REDUCING THE RISK OF CANCER

Recent evidence suggests that improved selenium nutrition may reduce the risk of cancer. Some of the best known studies on selenium were carried out by Dr Gerhard Schrauzer, Professor of Chemistry at the University of California. It was through Dr Schrauzer's research into breast cancer that he discovered the importance of selenium in the diet. His studies revealed that, although breast cancer is a universal disease, some populations of women have a lower risk of developing it than others. Japanese women, for example, have a much lower risk than American women. However, Japanese women who have emigrated to the United States are more at risk. The Japanese-American is also just as prone to the disease as the American.

Dr Schrauzer also discovered that Yugoslavian women have the same risk of developing breast cancer as Japanese women, although there are few links between the two countries. He examined the diet of both nations, first looking at how much meat and bread were being consumed. His initial discovery was that those with a higher standard of living were eating more meat and less bread and cereals. These people were more likely to develop cancer, so Dr Schrauzer worked on the hypothesis that eating meat and animal fat increases the probability that cancer will develop, while eating fish, bread and cereals reduces this risk.

He then began to examine the human diet, paying particular attention to trace elements and trace minerals. His research showed that the intake of selenium was the most variable factor around the world. In 1971, he discovered that one of the blood tests for cancer was also a test for the level of selenium in the blood and this forged the link between low levels of selenium and the risk of cancer. The next step was a major study to establish where selenium levels were low and how this related to the incidence of cancer. He and his colleagues found that, in twenty-seven countries, the cancer rate was inversely proportional to the dietary intake of selenium.

SELENIUM AND HEART DISEASE
There have been many trials involving selenium in the treatment of heart disease since it was discovered, in 1974, that it could cure Keshan's disease. This disease involves heart failure due to heart muscle weakness and it claimed the lives of many children and women of child-bearing age in China until selenium was used in

a trial involving over 1,000 Chinese children. Keshan's disease is more common in the large band of land running from the north-east to the south-west of China than anywhere else. This area has very low levels of selenium in the soil.

In the trial, selenium supplements were given to 4,510 children who had been selected at random. Another 3,980 were given a placebo and, after twelve months, the numbers in the groups were increased with 6,709 receiving extra selenium supplements and 5,445 being given the placebo, or dummy. The results were so impressive that the control group was abolished and all the 13,000 children involved were given selenium, bringing new hope and life to these communities. In 1976 there were only four cases of Keshan's disease and, twelve months after that, there were no new outbreaks of the disease in any of the 13,000 children being given selenium.

The most dramatic results with selenium have come from research based at The Cleveland Clinic in the US, where reports were collated from twenty-four countries concerning incidences of heart disease and the selenium content in the soil. This study revealed that Finland and the US, which are known to have some of the lowest levels of selenium, have more than four times as many instances of heart attacks as countries such as Yugoslavia, where the selenium content is one of the highest in the world.

SELENIUM AND FOOD

Research carried out by the Ministry of Agriculture, Fisheries and Food in 1977 showed that the total intake and amounts of selenium in major foods were low because of a low level of the element in British soil. Areas of North America, such as Wyoming and the Dakotas, have high levels of selenium in their soil, making their grain some of the most nutritious in the world.

Some parts of Europe are losing selenium from their soils at an alarming rate. In Sweden, the government is so concerned about the problem that they now offer a free daily supplement to all pregnant women. There is now concern that British soil is also falling below a safe standard: Norfolk, for example, used to have some of the highest levels of selenium in its soil, but these have been falling since the advent of intensive farming methods and the over-use of fertilisers. Studies show that, on average, our daily intake has dropped from 60mcg a day in 1975 to 35mcg today. This may be because, since joining the EU, we import a European wheat that is low in selenium, instead of the American grain that contains higher levels.

A substantial excess of selenium can cause birth defects, hair loss and blotchy skin. Selenium poisoning is unlikely to occur from our food but it may happen if too many supplements are taken. Government figures suggest that the maximum daily intake of selenium from all sources, including food, should not exceed 450mcg.

The level of selenium in food varies considerably depending on selenium levels in the soil. Cattle grazed on poor soil will not absorb much of the mineral from the grass and so will not contain much in their milk or meat. Likewise, eggs from chickens that have not been allowed to feed on selenium-rich foods will not contain as much as well-fed free-range birds. So buying free-range eggs is not only better for the birds, but can be of benefit to our bodies too. Brewer's yeast is also a good source of selenium and is especially useful for vegetarians and vegans. Other selenium-rich foods include wheat, shellfish, lentils, low-fat cheese, mushrooms, pasta and rice.

Selenium exists in various forms: organic selenium, best absorbed by the body, is included in some mineral supplements and is made by growing yeast in a selenium-enriched medium; inorganic selenium, such as sodium selenate, seems to be less easily absorbed by the body and is more toxic if taken in excess.

DAILY ALLOWANCE

Selenium is measured in micrograms (mcg). As yet, there is no RDA in Britain. However, it is thought that we need 1–2mcg for each kilo of body weight. The average adult weighing 70kg therefore requires a daily intake of 70–140mcg. The intake recommended by the World Health Organisation is 50–200mcg a day.

—5—

The New Antioxidants

Since research took off in the 1980s, more antioxidant nutrients
have been discovered and this has opened up a whole new area
of research. The 'new breed' of antioxidants are the flavonoids,
which are found in vegetables and herbs. There are over 4,000
flavonoid compounds altogether.

Fruit, vegetables and herbs contain a large number of non-
nutritive compounds, ie substances without apparent nutritive
value, but which have biological activity. Although scientists are
now convinced of the health-giving benefits of fruit and vegetables, they cannot be absolutely sure that it is down to one particular nutrient such as vitamin C or beta-carotene.

Flavonoids are an important group of non-nutritive
substances called polyphenols, which occur in foods of
vegetable origin. Recent in vitro and in vivo studies have
revealed that some flavonoids, particularly flavones and
flavonols, have a potentially protective effect against cancer and
coronary heart disease. Some flavonoids, principally those
found in high vitamin C foods, also help the body absorb and
utilise vitamin C – boosting its ability to act as an antioxidant
as well.

Flavonoids are found in most plants and there are many
different types: flavonols, flavones, flavonones, anthocyanidins,
catechins and bioflavons. To date over 4,000 different types of
flavonoids have been described and this number is increasing.

Flavonoids have several functions: they protect plants from
UV radiation, insects, fungi, viruses and bacteria. They also
control plant hormone levels and inhibit the activity of

certain enzymes. In foods, flavonoids may act as natural preservatives, although they impart a bitter flavour. It is due to this flavour that many flavonoids are removed from foods during processing.

It was originally thought that flavonoids had vitamin properties and, in the 1930s, they were known collectively as vitamin P. However, further research suggested that the claim that flavonoids were vitamins was not substantiated, and so the term vitamin P was abandoned in 1950. The importance of flavonoids in our diet is only recently being reassessed. It is still maintained that flavonoids show biological activities and so they have been awarded the title 'bioflavonoid'.

Flavonoids have a remarkable range of activities in humans, including free-radical scavenging. They can also inhibit many enzymes, a number of which are critically involved in the development of allergic and inflammatory disorders and even cancer. Other enzymes, which are involved in the development of retroviral diseases such as HIV-1 infection, can also be inhibited by certain flavonoids. Another benefit is their ability to adjust the functional activity of many types of cells including platelets, macrophages, lymphocytes, fibroblasts, smooth muscle, nerve and cancer cells. Certain flavonoids also appear to possess cholesterol-lowering effects and a recent study from the Netherlands showed an inverse correlation between the dietary flavonoid intake and the incidence of coronary heart disease.

Where to Find Flavonoids

Flavonols and flavones mainly occur in the leaves and outer parts of plants and only trace amounts are found in the underground part. One exception to this general rule is the onion, which contains a large amount of the flavonoid quercetin. In foods, flavonoids are usually bound to sugars such as glucose.

Dr Michael Hertog carried out an analysis of flavonoids in foods in the Netherlands with some interesting results. The study concentrated on the identification and the levels of five potential major anti-carcinogenic flavonoids in popular food. Dr Hertog noted that the levels of flavonoids in leafy vegetables such as lettuce, endive and leeks were influenced by the season. The levels were three to five times higher in summer than in other seasons – the formation of flavonoids is dependent on light. Growing plants in greenhouses also lowers the flavonoid content.

It is better to eat foods fresh as most methods of processing deplete the food of many nutrients. This is also true of flavonoids – levels in processed foods are generally 50 percent lower than in fresh products. However, if you are a fan of processed sweet cherries, bizarre as it may seem, these contain a higher level of the flavonol quercetin than fresh sweet cherries.

WINE AND TEA

Believe it or not, certain wines and teas contain flavonoids which may help prevent cancer and coronary heart disease. Food-derived flavonoids, such as quercetin, kaempherol and myricetin have been shown to inhibit cancerous tumours in rats and mice and the antioxidant flavonoids, primarily quercetin, prevent oxidation and reduce the risk of heart disease. It is even thought by some that the flavonoids in red wine are more powerful antioxidants than vitamin E. It is also remarkable that red wine can be diluted 1,000 times and still have an antioxidant activity comparable to that of 10µm quercetin. This startling fact has led investigators to attribute the low risk of heart disease in France to their high intake of red wine. The fact that the French eat a lot of fatty, greasy food and yet hardly suffer from coronary heart disease is referred to as 'The French Paradox'. Now that scientists have discovered antioxidants, it seems that the high intake of red wine and fresh fruit and vegetables in France is the key to their good health.

Beverages account for at least 25–30 percent of our daily flavonoid intake and Dr Hertog and his research team have reported on the flavonoid content of twelve types of tea, six types of wine and seven types of fruit juice.

The flavonoids myricetin and quercetin were found in red wines and grape juice (only one white wine analysed contained any flavonoids: a tiny level of myricetin). The highest flavonoid levels were found in Italian Chianti. Quercetin was found in fruit juice, with the highest amount in tomato juice. Interestingly, the level of quercetin in freshly squeezed orange juice was on a par with that of processed orange juice. Quercetin was also the most prominent flavonoid found in tea. Unfortunately, not all beverages contain flavonoids: beer and coffee contain no flavonoids at all and have virtually no health-giving properties.

Green tea has health benefits other than its antioxidant effect on the body. A report in the *Medical Tribune* in April 1992 remarked on the fact that compounds in this Japanese brew can kill *Streptococcus mutans*, a bacterium which can cause dental decay. The tannins in the tea are thought to halt the bacterium's production of glucans, which bind acid-generating bacteria to our teeth. We will, no doubt, be able to buy green tea toothpaste before too long.

In general, red wines are high in quercetin and myricetin. Fruit juices are quercetin-rich only (except for grape juice) and tea is high in quercetin and kaempherol.

In the Netherlands, tea is the main source of flavonoids (at 48 percent) and it is probably a similar figure in Britain; we each drink around 1,300 cups a year. Dr Hertog's research has sparked off many more studies throughout the world into the effect of tea in preventing cancer and heart disease. The American Heart Foundation claims that drinking up to ten cups of tea a day will give you the same amount of antioxidants as found in the recommended daily intake of fresh vegetables.

A team at Edinburgh University's cardiovascular research unit is, at the time of writing, in the final stages of a three-year study into the beneficial effects of tea in preventing heart disease. Tea also supplies half the average person's intake of manganese. However, tea also contains a lot of caffeine, an addictive stimulant, and tannin, which interferes with iron absorption. Further research is needed to establish just how much tea is good for us and in what form.

Flavonoids and Cancer

It was only very recently, in 1985, that it was discovered that quercetin inhibits the activity of carcinogens and scavenges the free radicals which are possibly involved in cell damage and the development of tumours. Recent studies show that some flavonoids, such as quercetin, inhibit carcinogenesis in rodents, and a study has now been carried out on humans; the Zutphen Elderly Study was published in *Nutrition and Cancer* in 1994. This assessed the flavonoid intake of 738 men aged sixty-five to eighty-four years, who had no history of cancer, and then studied them over a five-year period. Their main source of flavonoids was tea (at 61 percent) followed by fruit and vegetables: mainly onions, kale, endive and apples (38 percent). Between 1985 and 1990, seventy-five of the men developed cancer, and thirty-four died from cancer. Twenty-six men had a first diagnosis of lung cancer during this time. The study revealed that those who had a higher intake of flavonoids had a slightly lower risk of developing cancer. However, due to the small number of deaths from lung cancer, this association could not be substantiated and could merely be a chance finding.

The results clearly reveal a need for further epidemiological studies on the effects of flavonoids on cancer. It is interesting to note that the flavonoids in fruit and vegetables were associated with a lower risk of cancer, whereas the flavonoids in tea had no effect on cancer risk and, in fact, they tended to be associated with a higher risk of lung cancer. These results suggest that there are other constituents of fruit and vegetables, not present in tea, that are responsible for the lower cancer incidence rates. Alternatively, tea may contain other ingredients which enhance the risk of cancer. More studies are needed before the effect of flavonoids on cancer risk can be established.

Flavonoids and Heart Disease

Studies have shown that our arteries become clogged with cholesterol when lipoproteins, the fats which transport cholesterol in our blood, chemically combine with oxygen. The damaged lipoproteins are called *oxidised LDL*. Antioxidant nutrients protect us against heart disease by preventing LDL oxidation. It is now well known that oxidation occurs when the body is depleted of antioxidants. Vitamin E is our last defence against the free radicals that damage lipoproteins. However, our levels of vitamin E can be quickly destroyed during exposure to free radicals. Vitamin C then comes to the rescue by regenerating this 'spent' vitamin E. It is thought that flavonoids work synergistically with these antioxidants by boosting vitamin C, as well as possessing their own antioxidant properties.

The Zutphen Elderly Study also examined the relationship between flavonoid intake and the risk of coronary heart disease. Dietary and medical examinations were carried out on the elderly men in 1985 and again in 1990. Out of the 805 men involved in the study, 185 men had died, 43 of them from coronary heart disease. High intakes of flavonoids predicted a lower rate of mortality; coronary heart disease mortality was 60 percent lower in those men with a higher flavonoid intake. Quercetin was the predominant flavonoid in the diet.

It is also important to note that the major source of flavonoids in this study was tea, at 61 percent. There was a clear correlation between flavonoid intake and tea intake and both were associated with a lower risk of mortality from coronary heart disease. This may be due to substances in the tea other than flavonoids, such as antioxidant tea polyphenols. However, the effects of flavonoids on coronary heart disease mortality were stronger than the effect of tea alone.

Between 1958 and 1964, 12,763 men aged between forty and fifty-nine years enrolled in the Seven Countries Study, involving Finland, Greece, Italy, Japan, the Netherlands, the USA and Yugoslavia. The results of this large study revealed that the average flavonoid intake was inversely related with death from coronary heart disease. The link between the average flavonoid intake and death from lung cancer was weaker, although the results of the study also suggested that, the higher the intake of flavonoids, the lower the risk of lung cancer mortality. Flavonoid content was more strongly and positively linked with stomach cancer mortality.

The Future of Flavonoids

The few studies into flavonoids and disease prevention have had positive results, but larger epidemiological studies are needed. We know what the flavonoid content of many foods is, but there remains very little knowledge about how well humans absorb and utilise flavonoids. Until recently, the importance of flavonoids in our diet has been underestimated. We consume larger quantities of flavonoids in a balanced diet than we do vitamins C and E and beta-carotene. It is thought that flavonoids may be just as potent antioxidants as these nutrients.

It is now possible to buy many flavonoids as supplements. There is a patented blend of flavonoids, known as Pycnogenol, which is highly antioxidant and can be found on its own or in some good antioxidant supplements. Pycnogenol comes from the bark of the pine tree *Pinus maritima*, which is abundant in southern France. It was discovered and named by Professor Jacques Masquelier over twenty-five years ago. Four hundred years prior to this, the pine bark was being made into a tea as a cure for scurvy, due to its high vitamin C content.

Later analysis revealed that the extract was a concentrate of highly active flavonoids known as proanthocyanidins, which are powerful free-radical scavengers.

Rutin is a glycoside of quercetin and it is thought to strengthen and protect our capillaries and blood vessels. It is available as a supplement and many women take it to prevent the formation of broken blood vessels and varicose veins.

Herbal Remedy

The majority of herbs contain flavonoids and some are veritable cocktails of these and other antioxidant nutrients, including vitamin C and carotenoids. Herbs have been used since time began to treat an infinite variety of disorders. A number of herb essential oils have a proven antioxidant action. The antioxidative compounds are not necessarily found exclusively in the essential oil of the plant, but this is often the richest source of nutrients.

The following herbs have been demonstrated as having antioxidant activity: bay, bitter almond, calamus, celery, cinnamon, citronella, clove, laurel, lovage, mint, nutmeg, parsley, pepper, peppermint, pimento, rosemary, sassafras, spike and thyme. Many of these, such as bay, parsley, pepper and thyme, can be used in our cooking, not only to add flavour to our meals, but to boost our protection against free radicals as well. Other lesser known herbs, such as the leaves of the Ginkgo biloba tree, are also rich sources of antioxidant flavonoids. Ginkgo contains kaempherol and quercetin, among others, and research has revealed that it is highly effective in scavenging free radicals. It is widely used in France and Germany to improve blood flow and prevent arteriosclerosis (hardening of the arteries). Ginkgo is not part of our diet, but some antioxidant supplements contain the leaf extract.

One of the herbs that has attracted a great deal of interest recently is garlic. Clinical research and a small number of epidemiological studies suggest that garlic inhibits the development of cancer and helps to protect us against heart disease. Other members of the garlic family, such as onions and leeks, are currently under investigation to establish if they offer any protection against cancer.

It is thought that it is the antioxidant activity of garlic which provides protection from these diseases. Dr Arouma, at King's College London, has recently examined this activity in commercially available preparations of garlic and ginger. The ginger powder inhibited the peroxidation of phospholipids but the garlic was less effective, although both preparations could scavenge peroxyl and hydroxyl radicals. However, the antioxidant activity of these herbs needs to be put into perspective, as the levels of each herb used in the laboratory were higher than that which is likely to be consumed by humans. Nevertheless, while herbs may constitute a small part of our daily diet, they can help to boost the nutrient value of our meals and add a little extra protection against free radicals.

—— 6 ——
Active Anti-Ageing

The idea that antioxidant nutrients can slow down the ageing process is an exciting one. Most of us probably don't think much about growing older until our bodies begin to change – our system starts to slow down, we become less energetic, our vision blurs, our skin becomes wrinkled and our hair turns grey. Exactly what causes these changes is not yet clear, but it is now known that free-radical activity plays an integral part in the ageing process and their effect can be counteracted by antioxidant nutrients.

Basically, there are two types of ageing. The first is the natural, chronological state of growing older, which happens to us all. There is not a lot we can do to influence this, but if we are lucky, we can remain fit and active to the end of our lives.

The second type is premature degenerative ageing, wherein we develop diseases and conditions such as arthritis and cataracts. Nutritional science now offers us a chance to slow down premature ageing and improve the quality of our lives in old age. Our main adversaries in the ageing process are believed to be the free radicals. By helping to control these, we may be able to delay the onset of many diseases associated with ageing, including heart disease, cancer, Parkinson's disease and lowered immunity, and remain looking youthful by warding off the wrinkles.

Radical Tactics

Laboratory research confirms that when cells die, almost a third of their proteins are damaged beyond repair by free radical attack. According to the respected cancer researcher Dr Bruce Ames, each human cell receives at least 10,000 damaging 'hits' from free radicals every day. Normally, the body can repair the damage by using its own supply of enzymes and other proteins. But as we get older, this in-built ability to repair our cells is reduced. Fortunately, nature gives us an antidote in the form of the antioxidant vitamins. By eating more of these vitamins in everyday foods such as fruits, vegetables and wholegrains, we may be better equipped to enjoy our retirement.

Clinical trials are underway in many research centres around the world to prove that antioxidants do indeed extend human life. The interim reports are encouraging, but the final results will obviously not be available for some time. Meanwhile, research shows that the lifespan of an animal is directly related to its ability to repair free-radical damage.

Studies at the Scottish Agricultural College show that certain foods have the potential to delay the signs of ageing. Mice fed antioxidant extracts from plants and herbs have been found to live longer. Scientists examining the tissues of the mice found that those that had been fed regular amounts of antioxidants had healthier cells than those that had not received the nutrients.

Our cells are protected by essential fatty acids, but if we are exposed to too many free radicals the levels of these important acids drop dramatically. Dr Stanley Deans has been studying the effect of feeding thyme essential oil to mice. It was revealed that the animals that were fed thyme oil had higher levels of two important fatty acids than the other mice. One of these fatty acids, docosochexaenoic acid, was mainly found in the eyes of the treated mice. The level of this particular fatty acid usually declines with age and leads to loss of good eyesight. It may be that this can be counteracted in humans by boosting our intake of antioxidant herbs.

Other studies carried out in Germany indicate that feeding old rats with plant oils increases the release of an important neurotransmitter in their brains. Again, brain activity is something which usually decreases as we get older. Dr Deans explains:

> The beneficial effects of the antioxidants are profound because they have anti-ageing properties in animals. We may find, in the future, they help to reduce all kinds of ageing disorders, such as Alzheimer's disease and skin wrinkling.

Living Longer

Very few of us reach the ripe old age of 120, although this is an accepted lifespan for human beings. The vast majority of people will die prematurely from diseases. For other species, free radical damage is responsible for the ageing process, and now scientists are investigating whether this is true for humans also. Research on such varied creatures as lobsters and fruit-flies has revealed that low levels of free-radical activity dramatically increase life expectancy. In the case of the lobster and some of its marine companions, such as sea anemones, degenerative ageing appears not to be inevitable. It seems that these sea creatures are protected from free-radical damage in some way, and manage to grow old without deteriorating.

Earthly creatures, such as roundworms, are also protected from free radical attack by high levels of antioxidants in their system. Researchers at the University of Colorado have bred a strain of roundworm which enjoys a 65 percent increase in lifespan. These long-lived worms contain higher than normal amounts of antioxidants.

The idea of breeding species to extend their lifespan looks like becoming a reality in the not too distant future. According to Professor Michael Rose at the University of California, there is, for the first time:

*A real possibility of affecting the ageing process with bio-
medical intervention. There is nothing deeply problematic
about doubling the human lifespan. Ageing used to be mysteri-
ous and now it isn't. It is a problem that has been solved.*

Scientists at the University of California have bred fruit-flies
that can live for the equivalent of about 150 human years. The
genes of these flies contain the antioxidant SOD, which
neutralises free radicals and prevents cell damage.

Anti-Ageing Vitamins

The Americans are highly expert when it comes to researching
the ageing process. At the Human Nutrition Research Centre in
Boston, elderly volunteers check in for residual nutrition
programmes where every mouthful of food is monitored. The
research has shed a good deal of light on how antioxidant vitamins help to delay the ageing process. According to Professor
Jeffrey Blumberg, Associate Director, one of the most important findings is how the antioxidant vitamins boost our immune
systems.

Our immune system's responses slow down with age, but we
have found that vitamin E is very important in maintaining an
optimum immune response. High doses of vitamin E can stim-
ulate the immune system and may even regenerate it.

Some researchers suggest that the low levels of white blood
cells seen in the elderly are due to the life-long process of oxidation and production of free radicals. Beta-carotene has been
shown to boost the immune system and even reduce the size of
cancerous tumours in animals. There is strong evidence that
beta-carotene enhances many aspects of immunity and that a
diet rich in carotenoids is linked to a lower risk of developing
many types of cancer.

Other antioxidant nutrients have also been tested for their ability to boost the immune system. Research carried out by Professor Ranjit Chandra at the World Health Organisation for Nutritional Immunology tested the ACE vitamins on ninety-six healthy elderly volunteers. Two groups of individuals were involved in the trial. The first was given a daily dose of vitamins A, C, D and E, B-complex vitamins, beta-carotene, folic acid, iron, zinc, copper, selenium, iodine, calcium and magnesium. The quantities given were approximate to the RDAs, except for vitamin E and beta-carotene, which were given in much greater doses. The second group was given a dummy supplement containing only calcium and magnesium. Both groups took the supplements every day for twelve months. At the end of the trial, those who had taken the antioxidant supplements saw a 'significant improvement in several immune responses.' Professor Chandra concluded that, by taking vitamin supplements, we increase our immunity: 'Such an intervention led to a striking reduction in illness – a find that is of considerable clinical and public health importance.'

The evidence suggests that taking vitamin supplements does no harm and has enormous potential for controlling many crippling and costly chronic diseases. Professor Blumberg at the Human Nutrition Research Centre sums up by saying: 'I think we have enough data in hand for physicians to begin suggesting that patients take supplements, or at least not discourage them from it.' As he so aptly points out: 'No one seems to mind prescribing endless drugs for the elderly, so why not an inexpensive and safe nutrient?'

Cataracts

This condition is the world's number one cause of blindness and it mainly affects the elderly. As many as half the population aged seventy-five or over will suffer from this disorder, which causes a clouding of the eye lens and results in poor vision or even blindness in later life. The good news is that those in middle age who eat plenty of carrots, spinach and orange juice can dramatically reduce their risk. Beta-carotene, together with vitamins C and E, appears to slow down chemical changes in the eye lens.

When light is absorbed by the eye, it generates oxyradicals, a particularly active form of free radical. Oxyradicals appear to promote the formation of opacities on the lens – a type of protein that clouds the vision. The gelatine-like cells of the eyes, which are normally clear, become damaged, and tiny droplets of fat leak out. Oxyradicals also suppress the function of the enzymes that would normally get rid of these damaged proteins. These tiny particles block the vision and make the eyes look cloudy.

One study at the University of Western Ontario in Canada found that those who took vitamin E supplements averaging 400iu a day were half as likely to develop cataracts as those who did not. Those who took a mixture of both vitamins C and E cut their risk by two-thirds. Dr James Robertson, who conducted the Canadian trial, says that 'this information could have a large impact on the incidence of cataracts in older people.' As a follow-up study, he has been investigating an antioxidant cocktail, containing vitamins C and E and beta-carotene, as a way of protecting the eyes against the formation of cataracts. Interestingly, studies that dose patients with vitamin C lead to high levels of this vitamin being found in the eye lens, which indicates that the body sends it there to give some kind of protection.

The Brain Drain

One of the most distressing problems of old age is Alzheimer's disease. This tragic affliction causes the elderly to lose their memory, and become confused, dazed and disorientated. Sufferers have to be looked after every hour of the day and there is currently no way to improve their situation. There is no known cure for Alzheimer's disease and scientists are still a long way from pin-pointing its cause. However, French researchers have shown that some Alzheimer's sufferers have low levels of the antioxidant vitamins in their bloodstream. High levels of aluminium in the bloodstream is another popular theory, as aluminosilicate deposits are found in the brains of Alzheimer's sufferers. Scientists at the Dunn Nutrition Centre in Cambridge are investigating whether these deposits might involve free radicals.

Studies on the brain cells of mice have shown that free radicals and oxygen-derived metabolites are produced during the build-up of aluminium levels in the brain. Free radicals damage brain cells in much the same way as they do other cells in the body – they attack the fats that surround brain cells and disrupt delicate tissues. Autopsies on elderly people show that their brain cells are more damaged by oxidation from free radicals than are those in young people. It is not possible to carry out experiments on living human brain cells, so researchers turn instead to laboratory rodents for their research.

Scientists at the Oklahoma Medical Research Foundation have discovered that free radicals reduce the short-term memory of gerbils. This can be tested by putting gerbils in a small maze and recording how many mistakes they make as they attempt to find their way out. When elderly gerbils were placed in the maze they initially took twice as many wrong turnings as the younger gerbils, which had memorised their escape route. But, after doses of antioxidants, the elderly gerbils were able to leave the maze as quickly as the younger group. When the antioxidant treatment was stopped, the forgetfulness returned. This simple piece of research gives us hope that humans may also be able to overcome memory loss with the help of antioxidants.

Ginkgo biloba has recently attracted much scientific interest as a memory-boosting herb. The main active ingredients in Ginkgo are antioxidant flavonoids. Dr Desmond Corrigan of Trinity College, Dublin, has explained how it works:

By increasing the amount of blood going to the brain, ginkgo prevents the formation of dangerous free radicals. These occur when the brain is deprived of oxygen because of poor circulation, and ultimately cause the cells to die.

As yet there have been very few clinical trials involving this remarkable herb but, in 1987, Dr Keith Wesnes, at the University of Reading, ran trials measuring the effects of ginkgo on a panel of elderly patients. He discovered that, in memory tests, the herb significantly improved the reaction speeds of the patients as well as the accuracy of their answers. The potential of this herbal extract to prevent memory loss and even treat Alzheimer's disease is exciting and research into Ginkgo biloba continues.

Parkinson's Disease

Parkinson's disease is another crippling brain disorder that can strike at any age, but most often affects the middle-aged and elderly. Parkinson's disease stems from a malfunction of the brain cells that control movement. These cells produce a chemical called dopamine that is essential for the brain to send messages to muscles. As the brain cells die and dopamine levels drop, patients are left with trembling hands and limbs, a shuffling walk and an inability to control their actions. Although we do not know what causes these brain cells to die, some researchers believe that it may be due to oxidation and the action of free radicals.

The main drug used to treat Parkinson's disease is levodopa, which loses its effectiveness with prolonged use. For this reason, it is often best to delay drug treatment for as long as possible. Several studies have linked low levels of vitamin C with Parkinson's disease. With these two facts in mind, a study of the factors that cause the nerve cell degeneration seen in Parkinson's disease was carried out at the Neurological Institute of New York.

Patients with early signs of Parkinson's disease were advised to take high-dose supplements of vitamin E (3,200iu a day) and vitamin C (3,000mg a day). The patients were not yet taking levodopa, although they were taking other drugs in an attempt to delay levodopa therapy. A similar group of patients was managed in the same way, except that they did not receive the antioxidant vitamins. The time before levodopa became necessary was extended by two and a half years in the patients who were receiving the vitamins, as compared to those who were not. However, a recent follow-up study showed that vitamin E on its own was not effective, so the results are not conclusive.

Arthritis

Arthritis is another common affliction of the elderly. There are two basic forms of arthritis: the most frequent is osteoarthritis, and the less common is rheumatoid arthritis.

Osteoarthritis is a 'wear and tear' disorder of the joint cartilage, associated with changes in the underlying bone which cause joint problems. The hip, knee and thumb joints are mainly affected and it is a common affliction of athletes.

Rheumatoid arthritis is linked to damage to the immune system and is detected by a blood test, which shows the presence of the rheumatoid factor, and also by X-rays, which reveal changes around the affected joints. Less is known about rheumatoid arthritis, but it is thought to be linked to genetic disorders, diet and certain types of infection.

The term 'arthritic' is used to describe any kind of sore, stiff or aching joints. There may be several reasons why this soreness occurs, but the underlying cause in all cases is inflammation within the joints. The symptoms in each case are similar, too: pain, swelling, warmth, redness of the overlying skin, joint deformities and restricted mobility. One of the most important clues in seeking a cure for arthritis is the action of free radicals within the body. Internal inflammation is almost always triggered by free radical activity, so the theory is that antioxidant nutrients may be able to reduce or even prevent this.

Synovial fluid in the joints acts as a lubricant. When free radicals get into the synovial fluid they cause it to lose its lubricating properties by oxidising the fats in the fluid. Once it has been damaged in this way the synovial fluid is unable to lubricate the joints effectively and the result is severe inflammation.

Antioxidant nutrients may have an important role in neutralising the excess levels of free radicals that damage the synovial fluid. Many people with arthritis report that their symptoms subside if they switch to a wholefood diet that is rich in fresh fruits and vegetables and low in processed refined foods. The reason behind this may be that these foods are rich sources of antioxidants.

A study reported in *The Lancet*, in 1991, described how arthritic patients on a one-year vegetarian diet benefited from reduced swelling, greater mobility of the joints and a stronger grip. The special diet started with a week-long fast during which patients took only herbal teas, garlic, vegetable broth and juice extracts from carrots, beets and celery. After their fast, patients were put on an 'exclusion' diet, where foods were introduced one at a time to identify any allergic reactions. Wheat, citrus fruits, sugar and dairy products are all believed to provoke the symptoms of arthritis. To boost their frugal diet, the volunteers were given food supplements, including a daily dose of beta-carotene, vitamin C and vitamin E. At the end of the year, those who had made changes in their diet had greatly improved, while the control group, which made no changes, deteriorated. This study shows that those who boost their intake of antioxidant vitamins can improve their condition. Their increased levels of antioxidants are thought to have improved arthritis by keeping down the levels of free radicals in the synovial fluid and maintaining optimum movement.

War on Wrinkles

While the medical world has concentrated on life-threatening diseases, the cosmetic industry has been investigating the use of antioxidants for a more aesthetic purpose. The theory is that, if these vitamins help repair cells within the body, they should also be able to restore damaged skin cells on its surface. As a result, some of the jargon that was originally confined to biochemistry laboratories has been creeping onto the cosmetic counters. Pick up any jar of expensive facial cream and the chances are that it will mention free radicals and the skin-saving properties of vitamin E. But do these creams really make any difference to facial lines?

The skin's main function is to protect the body within and in doing so it comes under constant attack from free radicals. The main sources of such attack are sunlight and pollution. Free radicals actively damage the skin in several ways. They destroy the membranes surrounding the skin cells, causing the contents to leak out and disintegrate. They also encourage the breakdown of the collagen and elastin fibres that support the skin. Without this underlying support, the complexion slides, quite literally, downhill. The effects of gravity tend to pull the skin downwards and the action of free radicals within the skin encourages a visible loss of elasticity and tone. The antioxidant nutrients such as vitamin E and beta-carotene help mop up most of the free radicals linked to such destruction, while vitamin C is useful for stimulating the fibroblast cells to produce more collagen.

Vitamin E is thought to play a particularly important role in the protection against sun damage to the skin. Research has shown that vitamin E inhibits the oxidation of the fats in our skin cells. It is added to cosmetics as a natural moisturiser and has been demonstrated to have anti-inflammatory effects in animal and human studies. Further studies show vitamin E to be a potent wrinkle reducer and skin conditioner.

In a trial carried out over a four-week period, twenty women aged between forty-two and sixty-four years tested the effectiveness of a cream containing 5 percent natural vitamin E. The cream was applied daily to the corner of one eyelid, while the corner of the other eye was treated with a similar cream that did not contain any vitamin E. At the end of the month, an imprint of the skin was taken and a three-dimensional image made to show the depth of wrinkles surrounding each eyelid. More than half the women saw a visible improvement in the depth of their crow's feet after using the vitamin E cream. There was no discernible difference in the women who had the applications of plain cream. Researchers noted that the active cream encouraged a significant decrease in the length and depth of the wrinkles. The study concluded: 'When used in skincare products, natural vitamin E will protect the skin from ultra-violet light, reduce the appearance of fine facial lines and wrinkles, and help delay the progression of ageing.'

WRINKLE REDUCERS

Each of the antioxidant vitamins has great potential for keeping the complexion youthful, as they protect the cells in many different ways. In addition to outside influences, such as sunshine and pollution, our skin is also damaged by elements from within the body. As our skin ages, it becomes more susceptible to attack from certain enzymes, such as collagenase. This enzyme is encouraged by free radicals and can cut up and destroy collagen fibres, leading to wrinkles. Another enzyme that can damage the skin is elastase. This may destroy the elastin fibres in the skin, which leads to skin sagging and wrinkles. Both collagenase and elastase occur naturally and a certain amount is essential for strong, supple skin. However, their activity is increased by UV light and cigarette smoke. As we get older, we are more at risk, as it takes less sunlight to produce the high levels of enzymes that may damage the skin. Fortunately, vitamin C is involved with these enzymes and may help regulate their action within the skin.

However, it is difficult to add vitamin C to skin creams as it is easily oxidised and readily inactivated. Cosmetic scientists have found a way of coating molecules of vitamin C before adding them to a moisturiser, but this is time consuming and expensive. Beta-carotene is also being studied for inclusion in skin-care products, but the main problem is that it stains the skin yellow. For the time being, moisturising creams that contain vitamin C and E are the most promising for actually reducing the formation of fine lines and wrinkles. Using a vitamin-enriched moisturising skin cream delivers the antioxidants directly to the skin's surface where they form a protective buffer zone against environmental damage. Look for the words 'alpha tocopherol' among the ingredients, or squeeze the contents of a vitamin E capsule into a jar of your favourite product.

Taking regular doses of antioxidant nutrients internally is another way of protecting the skin, but the doses do need to be relatively high. This is because the transfer rate of vitamins from the liver to the skin is poor, as the nutrients are used up in other more important functions en route. Pycnogenol, the patented blend of antioxidant flavonoids, is also said to help to prevent the early facial wrinkles that occur due to skin inelasticity, when taken internally. Pycnogenol contains catechin flavonoids and studies at Baylor College of Medicine in Texas show that these bind tightly with skin collagen to protect it against the damage caused by enzymes. Pycnogenol also acts as an excellent sunscreen. Test-tube experiments carried out by Dr Antti Holevi Arstilla at the University of Jyvaeskylae in Finland revealed that, when human skin cells were exposed to UV radiation, Pycnogenol provided excellent protection – even better than equal amounts of vitamin E. In typical experiments of this type, sunlight will kill about 50 percent of the skin cells. However, when an adequate amount of Pycnogenol is added, about 85 percent of the skin cells survive. This is exciting news but, as yet, little research has been carried out into the antioxidant effects of Pycnogenol and it is not as widely available as vitamin E. However, it is found in many antioxidant supplements.

Supplements for a Radical Difference

While ageing is inevitable, the frailty, sickness and skin wrinkling that so often accompany it are not. No matter what our age, we can all boost our protection against free radical damage by ensuring that our diet is rich in antioxidant nutrients. For many years we have been told by nutritionists and doctors that if we eat a 'well-balanced diet' we do not need to take vitamin supplements. However, the extensive research carried out into antioxidants reveals that we may not be able to obtain the protective effect of these nutrients through our daily diet alone. In the past, advice for taking vitamins and minerals has been based on an RDA. This quantity is partly based on the amount of a nutrient necessary to prevent deficiency diseases. For example, vitamin C is needed to prevent scurvy, vitamin B1 to prevent beriberi and vitamin D to prevent rickets. What we do not yet know is how much these RDAs need to be increased to take into account the new-found antioxidant properties of some nutrients. According to Professor Diplock, one of the world's leaders in antioxidant research: 'The current recommendations for vitamin E and other antioxidants are inconsistent with actual human requirements for optimum nutrition.'

It is impossible to define RDAs for the antioxidant action of certain vitamins and minerals as there are no direct deficiency diseases, such as scurvy, involved. You do not die instantly from a shortage of vitamin E, although the long-term health implications may be serious. We are well aware of the minimum quantities of some vitamins needed to prevent deficiency diseases, but we do not know what level of these vitamins is needed to protect our cells from an excess of free radical activity. The million dollar question is this: what level of the antioxidant nutrients should we be receiving to prevent degenerative diseases such as cancer? For example, the European guidelines for vitamin E may be 10mg daily, but many of the studies of disorders such as heart disease have involved quantities in the order of 400iu (294mg) of natural vitamin E daily.

It is generally thought that it is better, health-wise, to get the vitamins we need through our diet and not by taking supplements. However, this is not as easy as it sounds, especially when the modern diet consists of mainly processed foods and not enough fresh fruit and vegetables. If you find it difficult to eat at least five portions of fruit and vegetables daily, then you will no doubt find it easier to reap the benefits of the antioxidant nutrients by taking them in supplement form.

It is also not necessarily the case that all nutrients are easier for the body to use when taken naturally in food as opposed to a supplement. A clinical trial carried out by the US National Cancer Institute revealed that more beta-carotene was found in the plasma of those who had been given a daily supplement of 12–30mg of beta-carotene, than was found in the blood of those who were given foods which are rich in beta-carotene, such as carrots and broccoli.

Vitamin E is particularly difficult to get in good amounts from our diet alone, as the foods in which it is found are so over-refined that much of the vitamin E is lost. Again, studies published in the *New England Journal of Medicine* have shown that the protective effect of vitamin E against heart disease was not derived from vitamin E in the diet, but from taking vitamin E supplements. Many senior researchers around the world are now recommending that we all take supplements of the antioxidant vitamins to promote better health.

Glossary

Antioxidant – a substance that prevents oxidation. Nutrients with antioxidant activity include beta-carotene, vitamin C and vitamin E.

Arteriosclerosis – damage to the main arteries due to a build-up of fatty deposits (especially cholesterol) that leads to heart disease.

Bioactive – how biologically active a substance is in the body.

Bioavailable – the extent to which the body can make biological use of a substance.

Carcinogen – a substance that causes cancer.

Cell membrane – the double layer of fatty material and proteins that surrounds each living cell of all organisms.

Cholesterol – a fatty substance that has many important functions throughout the body. Excess cholesterol may be deposited in the artery lining.

Degenerative disease – The loss of the capacity of cells, tissues and organs needed for the body to function normally.

DNA – Deoxyribonucleic acid, the basic material in the chromosomes of each cell containing the genetic code of life.

Enzyme – a substance produced by the body that regulates biochemical reactions.

Epidemiological studies – these look at the spread and risk of disease in large populations. Researchers gather vast amounts of information from tens of thousands of people to pick up patterns of disease in relation to diet, lifestyle or other factors.

Fibroblasts – a cell in connective tissue which is responsible for producing the precursors of collagen and elastic fibres.

Free radical – a reactive particle that contains one or more unpaired electrons, causing it to be highly unstable and sometimes destructive within the body. Free radicals are encouraged by exposure to pollutants such as cigarette smoke. They age cells by damaging their structure and DNA.

HDL – Abbreviation of *high-density lipoproteins*, the vehicles that transport excess cholesterol away from the arteries and return it to the liver for disposal.

LDL – abbreviation for *low-density lipoproteins*, the vehicles that carry fats around the body in the bloodstream. They are considered to be the 'bad' form of cholesterol as an excess can build up in the arteries and lead to arteriosclerosis.

Lipid – a technical name for any type of fat, oil or other fatty substance.

Lymphocytes – white blood cells which are involved in the immune system

Macrophages – a large scavenger cell present in connective tissue and many major organs and tissues, which is an important part of the body's immune system.

Molecules – organised groups of two or more atoms

Oxidation – the process of using oxygen to release energy from cells. Its side-effect is the production of free radicals.

Ozone – a form of oxygen in which three atoms of the element combine to form the molecule O_3. Ozone is a powerful oxidant and can produce free radicals when inhaled.

Placebo – a 'dummy' pill given to volunteers taking part in a blind clinical trial, in which participants do not know whether they are taking the active substance being tested or a placebo.

Platelets – disc-shaped structures in the blood which have several functions in arresting bleeding.

Protein – a family of molecules made by linking amino-acids together.

RDA – abbreviation of *recommended daily allowance*, the amount of vitamins and minerals needed to satisfy the needs of the population, as advised by governments.

Singlet oxygen – an active form of oxygen that can lead to free radical formation.

Superoxide dismatase – otherwise known as SOD. An antioxidant enzyme found naturally in cells within the body. One form of the enzyme contains manganese and the other contains copper and zinc. It plays an important part in the fight against free radicals.

Tumour – an abnormal swelling in the body, usually an abnormal growth of tissue. Cancerous tumours are life-threatening, while other tumours may be benign.

Useful Addresses

The Coronary Prevention Group
Plantation House
Suite 5/4
45 Fenchurch Street
London EC3M 3NN
Tel: 0171-626 4844

The Food Commission
3rd Floor
5–11 Worship Street
London EC2A 2BH
Tel: 0171-628 7774

Health Education Authority
Hamilton House
Mabledon Place
London WC1H 9TX
Tel: 0171-383 3833

Index

A

Ageing 6, 8, 17, 36, 59-74
anti-ageing and antioxidant nutrients 59-74
Alcohol 17-18, 43, 52-4
red wine 52-4
Alzheimer's Disease 61, 64-6
Antioxidant compounds *see* Flavonoids
Antioxidant minerals *see* Minerals, antioxidant
Antioxidant vitamins *see* Vitamins, antioxidant
Arthritis 8, 36, 42, 67-9

B

Bacteria 9, 50, 53
Beta-carotene 6-7, 11, 14-15, 24-31, 56, 62-4, 68-71, 73-5
and anti-ageing 62-4, 68-71
and cancer 27-8
and cataracts 64
definition of 25-7
and skin care 26, 69-71
Blood 7, 9, 13, 36, 41-2, 57-8, 62, 66
haemoglobin, production of 41-2

C

Cancer 6, 8, 14, 16-17, 21, 27-9, 33, 39, 44-6, 50-6, 58
and beta-carotene 27-8
and flavonoids 51-6, 58
of the skin 16-17
and selenium 44-6
and vitamin C 33
see also Smoking
Carotenoids 6-7, 11, 14-15, 24-31, 56, 62-4, 68-71, 73-5
Beta-carotene 6-7, 11, 14-15, 24-31, 56, 62-4, 68-71, 73-5
carotenoid composition of foods 29-30
Cataracts 6, 8, 63-4
Copper 6, 40-2, 77

D

DNA (deoxyribonucleic acid) 10-11, 75-6
Drugs, prescription 7

E

Enzymes 8-9, 11, 13, 40-1, 43, 50-1, 60, 71-2, 75, 77
antioxidant enzyme SOD 40, 77
Eyes 6, 8, 44, 63-4

F

Fats/lipids 11, 18-20, 55, 76
cooking oils 18-20
lipid peroxidation 11
lipoproteins 76
Flavonoids 18, 32-3, 50-8, 66, 71-2
Bioflavonoids 32-3
and cancer 51-6, 58
and heart disease 50, 52-6, 58
herbal remedies 57-8, 66
Free radicals 7-23, 26, 59-62, 65-6, 68-9, 71-2, 75-6
and ageing 59-62, 65-6, 68-9, 71-2
avoidance of pollutants 12-23
definition of 9, 75-6
and DNA 10-11
increased exposure to 9-10
Fruit 6, 22, 25-30, 32, 34-5, 37, 50, 54-5, 60, 73

G

Genetics 21

H

Heart disease 6, 8, 20, 33, 35-8, 44-7, 50, 52-6, 58, 73, 75
and flavonoids 50, 52-6, 58